Diabetic Prep For Beginners 2021

Diabetic Meal Prep For Beginners with Delicious And Comfortable Recipes. Enjoy A Healthy Lifestyle With Smart Diet Program.

TABLE OF CONTENTS

BREAKFAST RECIPES

Steel-Cut Oatmeal Bowl With Fruit And Nuts

Preparation time: 5 minutes

Cooking time: 20 minutes

Servings: 4

Ingredients:

- 1 cup steel-cut oats

- 2 cups almond milk

- ¾ cup water

- 1 teaspoon ground cinnamon

- ¼ teaspoon salt

- 2 cups chopped fresh fruit, such as blueberries, strawberries, raspberries, or peaches

- 1/2 cup chopped walnuts

- ¼ cup chia seeds

Directions:

1. In a medium saucepan over medium-high heat, combine the oats, almond milk, water, cinnamon, and salt. Bring to a boil,

—

reduce the heat to low, and simmer for 15 to 20 minutes, until the oats are softened and thickened.

2. Top each bowl with 1/2 cup of fresh fruit, 2 tablespoons of walnuts, and 1 tablespoon of chia seeds before serving.

Nutrition: calories: 288; total fat: 11g; saturated fat: 1g; protein: 10g; carbs: 38g; sugar: 7g; fiber: 10g; cholesterol: 0mg; sodium: 329mg

Whole-Grain Dutch Baby Pancake

Preparation time: 5 minutes

Cooking time: 25 minutes

Servings: 4

Ingredients:

- 2 tablespoons coconut oil

- 1/2 cup whole-wheat flour

- ¼ cup skim milk

- 3 large eggs

- 1 teaspoon vanilla extract

- 1/2 teaspoon baking powder

- ¼ teaspoon salt

- ¼ teaspoon ground cinnamon

- Powdered sugar, for dusting

Directions:

1. Preheat the oven to 400f.
2. Put the coconut oil in a medium oven-safe skillet, and place the skillet in the oven to melt the oil while it preheats.
3. In a blender, combine the flour, milk, eggs, vanilla, baking powder, salt, and cinnamon. Process until smooth.

---

4. Carefully remove the skillet from the oven and tilt to spread the oil around evenly.
5. Pour the batter into the skillet and return it to the oven for 23 to 25 minutes, until the pancake puffs and lightly browns.
6. Remove, dust lightly with powdered sugar, cut into 4 wedges, and serve.

Nutrition: calories: 195; total fat: 11g; saturated fat: 7g; protein: 8g; carbs: 16g; sugar: 1g; fiber: 2g; cholesterol: 140mg; sodium: 209mg

Mushroom, Zucchini, And Onion Frittata

Preparation time: 10 minutes

Cooking time: 20 minutes

Servings: 4

Ingredients:

- 1 tablespoon extra-virgin olive oil

- 1/2 onion, chopped

- 1 medium zucchini, chopped

- 11/2 cups sliced mushrooms

- 6 large eggs, beaten

- 2 tablespoons skim milk

- Salt

- Freshly ground black pepper

- 1 ounce feta cheese, crumbled

Directions:

1. Preheat the oven to 400f.
2. In a medium oven-safe skillet over medium-high heat, heat the olive oil.
3. Add the onion and sauté for 3 to 5 minutes, until translucent.

4. Add the zucchini and mushrooms, and cook for 3 to 5 more minutes, until the vegetables are tender.
5. Meanwhile, in a small bowl, whisk the eggs, milk, salt, and pepper. Pour the mixture into the skillet, stirring to combine, and transfer the skillet to the oven. Cook for 7 to 9 minutes, until set.
6. Sprinkle with the feta cheese, and cook for 1 to 2 minutes more, until heated through.
7. Remove, cut into 4 wedges, and serve.

Nutrition: calories: 178; total fat: 13g; saturated fat: 4g; protein: 12g; carbs: 5g; sugar: 3g; fiber: 1g; cholesterol: 285mg; sodium: 234mg

Spinach And Cheese Quiche

Preparation time: 10 minutes, plus 10 minutes to rest

Cooking time: 50 minutes

Servings: 4 to 6

Ingredients:

- Nonstick cooking spray

- 8 ounces yukon gold potatoes, shredded

- 1 tablespoon plus 2 teaspoons extra-virgin olive oil, divided

- 1 teaspoon salt, divided

- Freshly ground black pepper

- 1 onion, finely chopped

- 1 (10-ounce) bag fresh spinach

- 4 large eggs

- 1/2 cup skim milk

- 1 ounce gruyere cheese, shredded

Directions:

1. Preheat the oven to 350f. Spray a 9-inch pie dish with cooking spray. Set aside.

2. In a small bowl, toss the potatoes with 2 teaspoons of olive oil, 1/2 teaspoon of salt, and season with pepper. Press the potatoes into the bottom and sides of the pie dish to form a thin, even layer. Bake for 20 minutes, until golden brown. Remove from the oven and set aside to cool.
3. In a large skillet over medium-high heat, heat the remaining 1 tablespoon of olive oil.
4. Add the onion and sauté for 3 to 5 minutes, until softened.
5. By handfuls, add the spinach, stirring between each addition, until it just starts to wilt before adding more. Cook for about 1 minute, until it cooks down.
6. In a medium bowl, whisk the eggs and milk. Add the gruyere, and season with the remaining 1/2 teaspoon of salt and some pepper. Fold the eggs into the spinach. Pour the mixture into the pie dish and bake for 25 minutes, until the eggs are set.
7. Let rest for 10 minutes before serving.

Nutrition: calories: 445; total fat: 14g; saturated fat: 4g; protein: 19g; carbs: 68g; sugar: 6g; fiber: 7g; cholesterol: 193mg; sodium: 773mg

APPETIZER RECIPES

Sweet Potato and Roasted Beet Salad

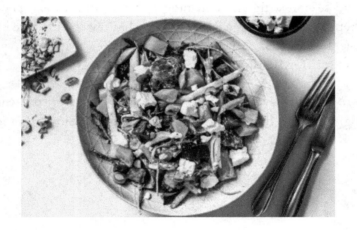

Preparation Time: 10 minutes,

Cooking Time: 10 minutes;

Servings: 4

Ingredients:

- 2 beets

- 1 sweet potato, peeled and cubed

- 1 garlic clove, minced

- 2 tablespoons walnuts, chopped and toasted

- 1 cup fennel bulb, sliced

- What you will need from the store cupboard:

  - 3 tablespoons balsamic vinegar

  - 1 teaspoon Dijon mustard

  - 1 tablespoon honey

  - 3 tablespoons olive oil

  - ¼ teaspoon pepper

  - ¼ teaspoon salt

  - 3 tablespoons water

Directions:

1. Scrub the beets. Trim the tops to 1 inch.
2. Wrap in foil and keep on a baking sheet.
3. Bake until tender. Take off the foil.
4. Combine water and sweet potato in a bowl.
5. Cover. Microwave for 5 minutes. Drain off.
6. Now peel the beets. Cut into small wedges.
7. Arrange the fennel, sweet potato and beets on 4 salad plates.
8. Sprinkle nuts.
9. Whisk the honey, mustard, vinegar, water, garlic, pepper and salt.
10. Whisk in oil gradually.
11. Drizzle over the salad.

Nutrition:

Calories 270, Carbohydrates 37g, Cholesterol 0mg, Fiber 6g, Sugar 0.3g, Fat 13g, Protein 5g, Sodium 309mg

Potato Calico Salad

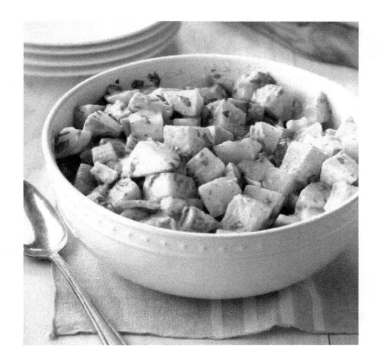

Preparation Time: 15 minutes,

Cooking Time: 5 minutes;

Servings: 14

Ingredients:

- 4 red potatoes, peeled and cooked

- 1-1/2 cups kernel corn, cooked

- 1/2 cup green pepper, diced

- 1/2 cup red onion, chopped

- 1 cup carrot, shredded

- What you will need from the store cupboard:

- 1/2 cup olive oil

- ¼ cup vinegar

- 1-1/2 teaspoons chili powder

- 1 teaspoon salt

- Dash of hot pepper sauce

Directions:

1. Keep all the ingredients together in a jar.

2. Close it and shake well.

3. Cube the potatoes. Combine with the carrot, onion, and corn in your salad bowl.

4. Pour the dressing over.

5. Now toss lightly.

Nutrition: Calories 146, Carbohydrates 17g, Cholesterol 0mg, Fiber 0g, Sugar 0g, Fat 9g, Protein 2g, Sodium 212mg

Mango and Jicama Salad

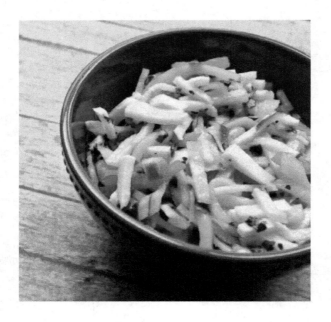

Preparation Time: 15 minutes,

Cooking Time: 5 minutes;

Servings: 8

Ingredients:

- 1 jicama, peeled

- 1 mango, peeled

- 1 teaspoon ginger root, minced

- 1/3 cup chives, minced

- 1/2 cup cilantro, chopped

- What you will need from the store cupboard:

- ¼ cup canola oil

- 1/2 cup white wine vinegar

- 2 tablespoons of lime juice

- ¼ cup honey

- 1/8 teaspoon pepper

- ¼ teaspoon salt

Directions:

1. Whisk together the vinegar, honey, canola oil, gingerroot, paper, and salt.

2. Cut the mango and jicama into matchsticks.

3. Keep in a bowl.

4. Now toss with the lime juice.

5. Add the dressing and herbs. Combine well by tossing.

Nutrition: Calories 143, Carbohydrates 20g, Cholesterol 0mg, Fiber 3g, Sugar 1.6g, Fat 7g, Protein 1g, Sodium 78mg

Asian Crispy Chicken Salad

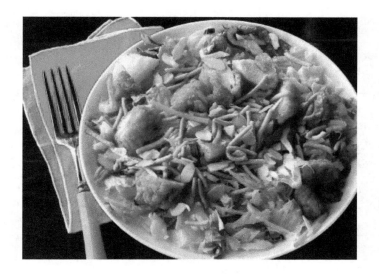

Preparation Time: 10 minutes,

Cooking Time: 10 minutes;

Servings: 2

Ingredients:

- 2 chicken breasts halved, skinless

- 1/2 cup panko bread crumbs

- 4 cups spring mix salad greens

- 4 teaspoons of sesame seeds

- 1/2 cup mushrooms, sliced

- What you will need from the store cupboard:

- 1 teaspoon sesame oil

- 2 teaspoons of canola oil

- 2 teaspoons hoisin sauce

- ¼ cup sesame ginger salad dressing

Directions:

1. Flatten the chicken breasts to half-inch thickness.

2. Mix the sesame oil and hoisin sauce. Brush over the chicken.

3. Combine the sesame seeds and panko in a bowl.

4. Now dip the chicken mix in it.

5. Cook each side of the chicken for 5 minutes.

6. In the meantime, divide the salad greens between two plates.

7. Top with mushroom.

8. Slice the chicken and keep on top. Drizzle the dressing.

Nutrition: Calories 386, Carbohydrates 29g, Cholesterol 63mg, Fiber 6g, Sugar 1g, Fat 17g, Protein 30g, Sodium 620mg

Kale, Grape and Bulgur Salad

Preparation Time: 10 minutes,

Cooking Time: 15 minutes;

Servings: 6

Ingredients:

- 1 cup bulgur

- 1 cup pecan, toasted and chopped

- ¼ cup scallions, sliced

- 1/2 cup parsley, chopped

- 2 cups California grapes, seedless and halved

- What you will need from the store cupboard:

- 2 tablespoons of extra virgin olive oil

- ¼ cup of juice from a lemon

- Pinch of kosher salt

- Pinch of black pepper

- 2 cups of water

Directions:

1. Boil 2 cups of water in a saùcepan

2. Stir the bulgur in and 1/2 teaspoon of salt.

3. Take out from the heat.

4. Keep covered. Drain.

5. Stir in the other ingredients.

6. Season with pepper and salt.

Nutrition: Calories 289, Carbohydrates 33g, Fat 17g, Protein 6g, Sodium 181mg

FIRST COURSE RECIPES

Cider Pork Stew

Preparation Time: 9 minutes

Cooking Time: 12 hours

Serving: 3

Ingredients

- 2 pounds pork shoulder roast

- 3 medium cubed potatoes

- 3 medium carrots

- 2 medium onions, sliced

- 1 cup coarsely chopped apple

- ½ cup coarsely chopped celery

- 3 tablespoons quick-cooking tapioca

- 2 cups apple juice

- 1 teaspoon salt

- 1 teaspoon caraway seeds

- ¼ teaspoon black pepper

Direction

1. Chop the meat into 1-in. cubes. In the 3.5- 5.5 qt. slow cooker, mix the tapioca, celery, apple, onions, carrots, potatoes and meat. Whisk in pepper, caraway seeds, salt and apple juice.

2. Keep covered and cook over low heat setting for 10-12 hours. If you want, use the celery leaves to decorate each of the servings.

Nutrition 244 Calories 5g Fiber 33g Carbohydrate

Creamy Chicken Noodle Soup

Preparation Time: 7 minutes

Cooking Time: 8 hours

Serving: 4

Ingredients

- 1 (32 fluid ounce) container reduced-sodium chicken broth

- 3 cups water

- 2½ cups chopped cooked chicken

- 3 medium carrots, sliced

- 3 stalks celery

- 1½ cups sliced fresh mushrooms

- ¼ cup chopped onion

- 1½ teaspoons dried thyme, crushed

- ¾ teaspoon garlic-pepper seasoning

- 3 ounces reduced-fat cream cheese (Neufchâtel), cut up

- 2 cups dried egg noodles

Direction

1. Mix together the garlic-pepper seasoning, thyme, onion, mushrooms, celery, carrots, chicken, water and broth in a 5 to 6-quart slow cooker.

2. Put cover and let it cook for 6-8 hours on low-heat setting.

3. Increase to high-heat setting if you are using low-heat setting. Mix in the cream cheese until blended. Mix in uncooked noodles. Put cover and let it cook for an additional 20-30 minutes or just until the noodles become tender.

Nutrition 170 Calories 3g Sugar 2g Fiber

Cuban Pulled Pork Sandwich

Preparation Time: 6 minutes

Cooking Time: 5 hours

Serving: 5

Ingredients

- 1 teaspoon dried oregano, crushed

- ¾ teaspoon ground cumin

- ½ teaspoon ground coriander

- ¼ teaspoon salt

- ¼ teaspoon black pepper

- ¼ teaspoon ground allspice

- 1 2 to 2½-pound boneless pork shoulder roast

- 1 tablespoon olive oil

- Nonstick cooking spray

- 2 cups sliced onions

- 2 green sweet peppers, cut into bite-size strips

- ½ to 1 fresh jalapeño pepper

- 4 cloves garlic, minced

- ¼ cup orange juice

- ¼ cup lime juice

- 6 heart-healthy wheat hamburger buns, toasted

- 2 tablespoons jalapeño mustard

Direction

1. Mix allspice, oregano, black pepper, cumin, salt, and coriander together in a small bowl. Press each side of the roast into the spice mixture. On medium-high heat, heat oil in a big non-stick pan; put in roast. Cook for 5mins until both sides of the roast is light brown, turn the roast one time.

2. Using a cooking spray, grease a 3 1/2 or 4qt slow cooker; arrange the garlic, onions, jalapeno, and green peppers in a layer. Pour in lime juice and orange juice. Slice the roast if needed to fit inside the cooker; put on top of the vegetables covered or 4 1/2-5hrs on high heat setting.

3. Move roast to a cutting board using a slotted spoon. Drain the cooking liquid and keep the jalapeno, green peppers, and onions. Shred the roast with 2 forks then place it back in the cooker. Remove fat from the liquid. Mix half cup of cooking liquid and reserved vegetables into the cooker. Pour in more cooking liquid if desired. Discard the remaining cooking liquid.

4. Slather mustard on rolls. Split the meat between the bottom roll halves. Add avocado on top if desired. Place the roll tops to sandwiches.

Nutrition 379 Calories 32g Carbohydrate 4g Fiber

SECOND COURSE RECIPES

Pasta Salad

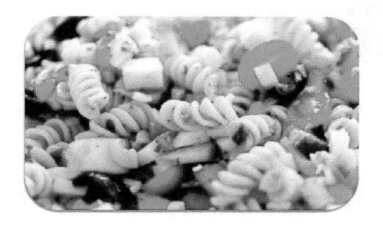

Preparation Time: 15 Minutes

Cooking Time: 15 Minutes

Servings: 4

Ingredients

- 8 oz. whole-wheat pasta

- 2 tomatoes

- 1 (5-oz) pkg spring mix

- 9 slices bacon

- 1/3 cup mayonnaise (reduced-fat)

- 1 tbsp. Dijon mustard

- 3 tbsp. apple cider vinegar

- 1/4 tsp. salt

- 1/2 tsp. pepper

Directions

1. Cook pasta.

2. Chilled pasta, chopped tomatoes and spring mix in a bowl.

3. Crumble cooked bacon over pasta.

4. Combine mayonnaise, mustard, vinegar, salt and pepper in a small bowl.

5. Pour dressing over pasta, stirring to coat.

Nutrition: Calories 200 / Protein 15 g / Fat 3 g / Carbs 6 g

Chicken, Strawberry, And Avocado Salad

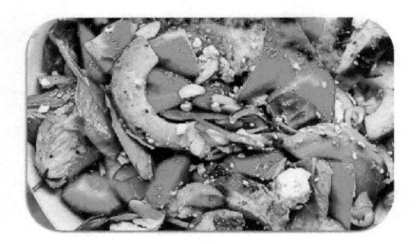

Preparation Time: 10 Minutes

Cooking Time: 5 Minutes

Ingredients

- 1,5 cups chicken (skin removed)

- 1/4 cup almonds

- 2 (5-oz) pkg salad greens

- 1 (16-oz) pkg strawberries

- 1 avocado

- 1/4 cup green onion

- 1/4 cup lime juice

- 3 tbsp. extra virgin olive oil

- 2 tbsp. honey

- 1/4 tsp. salt

- 1/4 tsp. pepper

Directions

1. Toast almonds until golden and fragrant.

2. Mix lime juice, oil, honey, salt, and pepper.

3. Mix greens, sliced strawberries, chicken, diced avocado, and sliced green onion and sliced almonds; drizzle with dressing. Toss to coat.

Nutrition: Calories 150 / Protein 15 g / Fat 10 g / Carbs 5 g

Lemon-Thyme Eggs

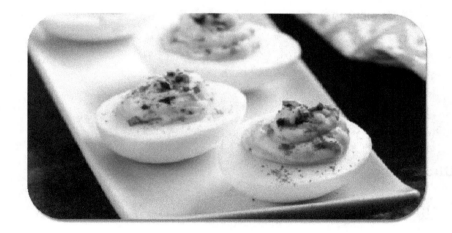

Preparation Time: 10 Minutes

Cooking Time: 5 Minutes

Servings: 4

Ingredients

- 7 large eggs

- 1/4 cup mayonnaise (reduced-fat)

- 2 tsp. lemon juice

- 1 tsp. Dijon mustard

- 1 tsp. chopped fresh thyme

- 1/8 tsp. cayenne pepper

Directions

1. Bring eggs to a boil.

2. Peel and cut each egg in half lengthwise.

3. Remove yolks to a bowl. Add mayonnaise, lemon juice, mustard, thyme, and cayenne to egg yolks; mash to blend. Fill egg white halves with yolk mixture.

4. Chill until ready to serve.

Nutrition: Calories 40 / Protein 10 g / Fat 6 g / Carbs 2 g

Spinach Salad with Bacon

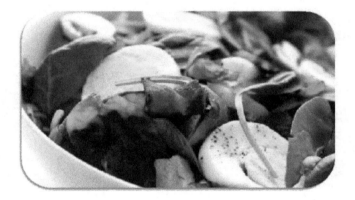

Preparation Time: 15 Minutes

Cooking Time: 0 Minutes

Servings: 4

Ingredients

- 8 slices center-cut bacon

- 3 tbsp. extra virgin olive oil

- 1 (5-oz) pkg baby spinach

- 1 tbsp. apple cider vinegar

- 1 tsp. Dijon mustard

- 1/2 tsp. honey

- 1/4 tsp. salt

- 1/2 tsp. pepper

Directions

1. Mix vinegar, mustard, honey, salt and pepper in a bowl.

2. Whisk in oil. Place spinach in a serving bowl; drizzle with dressing, and toss to coat.

3. Sprinkle with cooked and crumbled bacon.

Nutrition: Calories 110 / Protein 6 g / Fat 2 g / Carbs 1 g

Pea and Collards Soup

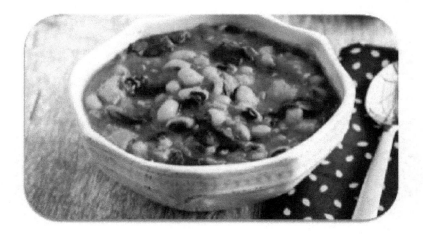

Preparation Time: 10 Minutes

Cooking Time: 50 Minutes

Servings: 4

Ingredients

- 1/2 (16-oz) pkg black-eyed peas

- 1 onion

- 2 carrots

- 1,5 cups ham (low-sodium)

- 1 (1-lb) bunch collard greens (trimmed)

- 1 tbsp. extra virgin olive oil

- 2 cloves garlic

- 1/2 tsp. black pepper

- Hot sauce

Directions

1. Cook chopped onion and carrots 10 Minutes.

2. Add peas, diced ham, collards, and Minced garlic. Cook 5 Minutes.

3. Add broth, 3 cups water, and pepper. Bring to a boil; simmer 35 Minutes, adding water if needed.

Nutrition: Calories 86 / Protein 15 g / Fat 2 g / Carbs 9 g

SIDE DISH RECIPES

Pinto Beans

Preparation Time: 6 minutes

Cooking Time: 55 minutes

Servings: 10

Ingredients:

- 2 cups pinto beans, dried

- 1 medium white onion

- 1 ½ teaspoon minced garlic

- ¾ teaspoon salt

- 1/4 teaspoon ground black pepper

- 1 teaspoon red chili powder

- 1/4 teaspoon cumin

- 1 tablespoon olive oil

- 1 teaspoon chopped cilantro

- 5 ½ cup vegetable stock

Directions:

1. 1.Plugin instant pot, insert the inner pot, press sauté/simmer button, add oil and when hot, add onion and garlic and cook for 3 minutes or until onions begin to soften.
2. 2.Add remaining ingredients, stir well, then press the cancel button, shut the instant pot with its lid and seal the pot.
3. 3.Click 'manual' button, then press the 'timer' to set the cooking time to 45 minutes and cook at high pressure.
4. 4.Once done, click 'cancel' button and do natural pressure release for 10 minutes until pressure nob drops down.
5. 5.Open the instant pot, spoon beans into plates and serve.

Nutrition: 107 Calories 11.7g Carbohydrates 4g Fiber

Parmesan Cauliflower Mash

Preparation Time: 19 minutes

Cooking Time: 5 minutes

Servings: 4

Ingredients:

- 1 head cauliflower

- ½ teaspoon kosher salt

- ½ teaspoon garlic pepper

- 2 tablespoons plain Greek yogurt

- ¾ cup freshly grated Parmesan cheese

- 1 tablespoon unsalted butter or ghee (optional)

- Chopped fresh chives

Directions:

1. 1.Pour cup of water into the electric pressure cooker and insert a steamer basket or wire rack.
2. 2.Place the cauliflower in the basket.
3. 3.Cover lid of the pressure cooker to seal.
4. 4.Cook on high pressure for 5 minutes.
5. 5.Once complete, hit Cancel and quick release the pressure.
6. 6.When the pin drops, remove the lid.
7. 7.Remove the cauliflower from the pot and pour out the water. Return the cauliflower to the pot and add the salt, garlic pepper,

yogurt, and cheese. Use an immersion blender to purée or mash the cauliflower in the pot.

8. 8.Spoon into a serving bowl, and garnish with butter (if using) and chives.

Nutrition: 141 Calories 12g Carbohydrates 4g Fiber

Steamed Asparagus

Preparation Time: 3 minutes

Cooking Time: 2 minutes

Servings: 4

Ingredients:

- 1 lb. fresh asparagus, rinsed and tough ends trimmed

- 1 cup water

Direction:

1. 1.Place the asparagus into a wire steamer rack, and set it inside your Instant Pot.
2. 2.Add water to the pot. Close and seal the lid, turning the steam release valve to the "Sealing" position.
3. 3.Select the "Steam" function to cook on high pressure for 2 minutes.
4. 4.Once done, do a quick pressure release of the steam.
5. 5.Lift the wire steamer basket out of the pot and place the asparagus onto a serving plate.
6. 6.Season as desired and serve.

Nutrition: 22 Calories 4g Carbohydrates 2g Protein

Squash Medley

Preparation Time: 10 minutes

Cooking Time: 20 minutes.

Servings: 2

Ingredients:

- 2 lbs. mixed squash

- ½ cup mixed veg

- 1 cup vegetable stock

- 2 tbsps. olive oil

- 2 tbsps. mixed herbs

Direction:

1. 1.Put the squash in the steamer basket and add the stock into the Instant Pot.
2. 2.Steam the squash in your Instant Pot for 10 minutes.
3. 3.Depressurize and pour away the remaining stock.
4. 4.Set to sauté and add the oil and remaining ingredients.
5. 5.Cook until a light crust form.

Nutrition: 100 Calories 10g Carbohydrates 6g Fat

SOUP & STEW

Swiss Cauliflower-Omental-Soup

Preparation time: 10 minutes

Cooking time: 15 minutes

Servings: 3-4

Ingredients:

- 2 cups cauliflower pieces

- 1 cup potatoes, cubed

- 2 cups vegetables stock (without yeast)

- 3 tbsp. Swiss Omental cheddar, cubed

- 2 tbsp. new chives

- 1 tbsp. pumpkin seeds

- 1 touch of nutmeg and cayenne pepper

Directions:

1. Cook cauliflower and potato in vegetable stock until delicate and Blend with a blender.

2. Season the soup with nutmeg and cayenne, and possibly somewhat salt and pepper.

3. Include Emmenthal cheddar and chives and mix a couple of moments until the soup is smooth and prepared to serve. Enhance it with pumpkin seeds.

Nutrition: Calories: 65 Carbohydrates: 13g Fat: 2g Protein: 1g

Chilled Parsley-Gazpacho with Lime & Cucumber

Preparation time: 10 minutes

Cooking time: 2 hours

Servings: 1

Ingredients:

- 4-5 middle sized tomatoes

- 2 tbsp. olive oil, extra virgin and cold pressed

- 2 large cups fresh parsley

- 2 ripe avocados

- 2 cloves garlic, diced

- 2 limes, juiced

- 4 cups vegetable broth

- 1 middle sized cucumber

- 2 small red onions, diced

- 1 tsp. dried oregano

- 1½ tsp. paprika powder

- ½ tsp. cayenne pepper

- Sea salt and freshly ground pepper to taste

Directions:

1. In a pan, heat up olive oil and sauté onions and garlic until translucent. Set aside to cool down.

2. Use a large blender and blend parsley, avocado, tomatoes, cucumber, vegetable broth, lime juice and onion-garlic mix until smooth. Add some water if desired, and season with cayenne pepper, paprika powder, oregano, salt and pepper. Blend again and put in the fridge for at least 1, 5 hours.

3. Tip: Add chives or dill to the gazpacho. Enjoy this great alkaline (cold) soup!

Nutrition: Calories: 48 Carbohydrates: 12 g Fat: 0.8g

Chilled Avocado Tomato Soup

Preparation time: 7 minutes

Cooking time: 20 minutes

Servings: 1-2

Ingredients:

- 2 small avocados

- 2 large tomatoes

- 1 stalk of celery

- 1 small onion

- 1 clove of garlic

- Juice of 1 fresh lemon

- 1 cup of water (best: alkaline water)

- A handful of fresh lavages

- Parsley and sea salt to taste

Directions:

1. Scoop the avocados and cut all veggies in little pieces.

2. Spot all fixings in a blender and blend until smooth.

3. Serve chilled and appreciate this nutritious and sound soluble soup formula!

Nutrition: Calories: 68 Carbohydrates: 15g Fat: 2g Protein: .8g

Pumpkin and White Bean Soup with Sage

Preparation time: 10 minutes

Cooking time: 40 minutes

Servings: 3-4

Ingredients:

- 1 ½ pound pumpkin

- ½ pound yams

- ½ pound white beans

- 1 onion

- 2 cloves of garlic

- 1 tbsp. of cold squeezed additional virgin olive oil

- 1 tbsp. of spices (your top picks)

- 1 tbsp. of sage

- 1 ½ quart water (best: antacid water)

- A spot of ocean salt and pepper

Directions:

1. Cut the pumpkin and potatoes in shapes, cut the onion and cut the garlic, the spices and the sage in fine pieces.

61

2. Sauté the onion and also the garlic in olive oil for around two or three minutes.

3. Include the potatoes, pumpkin, spices and sage and fry for an additional 5 minutes.

4. At that point include the water and cook for around 30 minutes (spread the pot with a top) until vegetables are delicate.

5. At long last include the beans and some salt and pepper. Cook for an additional 5 minutes and serve right away. Prepared!! Appreciate this antacid soup. Alkalizing tasty!

Nutrition: Calories: 78 Carbohydrates: 12g

Alkaline Carrot Soup with Millet

Preparation time: 7 minutes

Cooking time: 40 minutes

Servings: 3-4

Ingredients:

- 2 cups cauliflower pieces

- 1 cup potatoes, cubed

- 2 cups vegetables stock (without yeast)

- 3 tbsp. Swiss Emmenthal cheddar, cubed

- 2 tbsp. new chives

- 1 tbsp. pumpkin seeds

- 1 touch of nutmeg and cayenne pepper

Directions:

1. Cook cauliflower and potato in vegetable stock until delicate and Blend with a blender.

2. Season the soup with nutmeg and cayenne, and possibly somewhat salt and pepper.

3. Include Emmenthal cheddar and chives and mix a couple of moments until the soup is smooth and prepared to serve. Can enhance with pumpkin seeds.

Nutrition: Calories: 65 Carbohydrates: 15g Fat: 1g Protein: 2g

DESSERT

Cheese Cake

Preparation Time: 15 minutes

Cooking Time: 50 minutes

Servings: 6

Ingredients:

For Almond Flour Cheesecake Crust:

- 2 Cups of Blanched almond flour

- 1/3 Cup of almond Butter

- 3 Tablespoons of Erythritol (powdered or granular)

- 1 Teaspoon of Vanilla extract

For Keto Cheesecake Filling:

- 32 Oz of softened Cream cheese

- 1 and ¼ cups of powdered erythritol

- 3 Large Eggs

- 1 Tablespoon of Lemon juice

- 1 Teaspoon of Vanilla extract

Directions:

1. 1.Preheat your oven to a temperature of about 350 degrees F.
2. 2.Grease a spring form pan of 9" with cooking spray or just line its bottom with a parchment paper.
3. 3.In order to make the cheesecake rust, stir in the melted butter, the almond flour, the vanilla extract and the erythritol in a large bowl.
4. 4.The dough will get will be a bit crumbly; so, press it into the bottom of your prepared tray.
5. 5.Bake for about 12 minutes; then let cool for about 10 minutes.
6. 6.In the meantime, beat the softened cream cheese and the powdered sweetener at a low speed until it becomes smooth.
7. 7.Crack in the eggs and beat them in at a low to medium speed until it becomes fluffy. Make sure to add one a time.
8. 8.Add in the lemon juice and the vanilla extract and mix at a low to medium speed with a mixer.
9. 9.Pour your filling into your pan right on top of the crust. You can use a spatula to smooth the top of the cake.
10. 10.Bake for about 45 to 50 minutes.
11. 11.Remove the baked cheesecake from your oven and run a knife around its edge.
12. 12.Let the cake cool for about 4 hours in the refrigerator.
13. 13.Serve and enjoy your delicious cheese cake!

Nutrition 325 Calories 6g Carbohydrates 1g Fiber

Orange Cake

Preparation Time: 10 minutes

Cooking Time: 50minutes

Servings: 8

Ingredients:

- 2 and ½ cups of almond flour

- 2 Unwaxed washed oranges

- 5 Large separated eggs

- 1 Teaspoon of baking powder

- 2 Teaspoons of orange extract

- 1 Teaspoon of vanilla bean powder

- 6 Seeds of cardamom pods crushed

- 16 drops of liquid stevia; about 3 teaspoons

- 1 Handful of flaked almonds to decorate

Directions:

1. 1.Preheat your oven to a temperature of about 350 Fahrenheit.
2. 2.Line a rectangular bread baking tray with a parchment paper.
3. 3.Place the oranges into a pan filled with cold water and cover it with a lid.

4. 4.Bring the saucepan to a boil, then let simmer for about 1 hour and make sure the oranges are totally submerged.
5. 5.Make sure the oranges are always submerged to remove any taste of bitterness.
6. 6.Cut the oranges into halves; then remove any seeds; and drain the water and set the oranges aside to cool down.
7. 7.Cut the oranges in half and remove any seeds, then puree it with a blender or a food processor.
8. 8.Separate the eggs; then whisk the egg whites until you see stiff peaks forming.
9. 9.Add all your ingredients except for the egg whites to the orange mixture and add in the egg whites; then mix.
10. 10.Pour the batter into the cake tin and sprinkle with the flaked almonds right on top.
11. 11.Bake your cake for about 50 minutes.
12. 12.Remove the cake from the oven and set aside to cool for 5 minutes.

Nutrition 164 Calories 7.1g Carbohydrates 2.7g Fiber

Madeleine

Preparation Time: 10 minutes

Cooking Time: 15 minutes

Servings: 12

Ingredients

- 2 Large pastured eggs

- ¾ Cup of almond flour

- 1 and ½ Tablespoons of Swerve

- ¼ Cup of cooled, melted coconut oil

- 1 Teaspoon of vanilla extract

- 1 Teaspoon of almond extract

- 1 Teaspoon of lemon zest

- ¼ Teaspoon of salt

Directions

1. 1.Preheat your oven to a temperature of about 350 F.
2. 2.Combine the eggs with the salt and whisk on a high speed for about 5 minutes.
3. 3.Slowly add in the Swerve and keep mixing on high for 2 additional minutes.
4. 4.Stir in the almond flour until it is very well-incorporated; then add in the vanilla and the almond extracts.
5. 5.Add in the melted coconut oil and stir all your ingredients together.
6. 6.Pour the obtained batter into equal parts in a greased Madeleine tray.
7. 7.Bake your Ketogenic Madeleine for about 13 minutes or until the edges start to have a brown color.
8. 8.Flip the Madeleines out of the baking tray.

Nutrition 87 Calories 3g Carbohydrates 3g Fiber

Waffles

Preparation Time: 20 minutes

Cooking Time: 30 minutes

Servings: 3

Ingredients:

For Ketogenic waffles:

- 8 Oz of cream cheese

- 5 Large pastured eggs

- 1/3 Cup of coconut flour

- ½ Teaspoon of Xanthan gum

- 1 Pinch of salt

- ½ Teaspoon of vanilla extract

- 2 Tablespoons of Swerve

- ¼ Teaspoon of baking soda

- 1/3 Cup of almond milk

Optional ingredients:

- ½ Teaspoon of cinnamon pie spice

- ¼ Teaspoon of almond extract

For low-carb Maple Syrup:

- 1 Cup of water

- 1 Tablespoon of Maple flavor

- ¾ Cup of powdered Swerve

- 1 Tablespoon of almond butter

- ½ Teaspoon of Xanthan gum

Directions

1. For the waffles:
2. 1.Make sure all your ingredients are exactly at room temperature.
3. 2.Place all your ingredients for the waffles from cream cheese to pastured eggs, coconut flour, Xanthan gum, salt, vanilla extract, the Swerve, the baking soda and the almond milk except for the almond milk with the help of a processor.
4. 3.Blend your ingredients until it becomes smooth and creamy; then transfer the batter to a bowl.
5. 4.Add the almond milk and mix your ingredients with a spatula.
6. 5.Heat a waffle maker to a temperature of high.
7. 6.Spray your waffle maker with coconut oil and add about ¼ of the batter in it evenly with a spatula into your waffle iron.
8. 7.Close your waffle and cook until you get the color you want.
9. 8.Carefully remove the waffles to a platter.
10. For the Ketogenic Maple Syrup:
11. 9.Place 1 and ¼ cups of water, the swerve and the maple in a small pan and bring to a boil over a low heat; then let simmer for about 10 minutes.
12. 10.Add the coconut oil.
13. 11.Sprinkle the Xanthan gum over the top of the waffle and use an immersion blender to blend smoothly.
14. 12.Serve and enjoy your delicious waffles!

Nutrition 316 Calories 7g Carbohydrates 3g Fiber

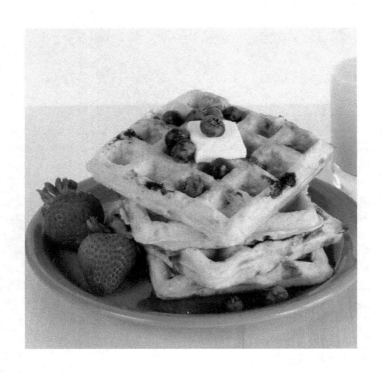

Pretzels

Preparation Time: 10 minutes

Cooking Time: 20 minutes

Servings: 8

Ingredients:

- 1 and ½ cups of pre-shredded mozzarella

- 2 Tablespoons of full fat cream cheese

- 1 Large egg

- ¾ Cup of almond flour+ 2 tablespoons of ground almonds or almond meal

- ½ Teaspoon of baking powder

- 1 Pinch of coarse sea salt

Directions:

1. 1.Heat your oven to a temperature of about 180 C/356 F.
2. 2.Melt the cream cheese and the mozzarella cheese and stir over a low heat until the cheeses are perfectly melted.
3. 3.If you choose to microwave the cheese, just do that for about 1 minute no more and if you want to do it on the stove, turn off the heat as soon as the cheese is completely melted.
4. 4.Add the large egg to the prepared warm dough; then stir until your ingredients are very well combined. If the egg is cold; you will need to heat it gently.

5. 5.Add in the ground almonds or the almond flour and the baking powder and stir until your ingredients are very well combined.
6. 6.Take one pinch of the dough of cheese and toll it or stretch it in your hands until it is about 18 to 20 cm of length; if your dough is sticky, you can oil your hands to avoid that.
7. 7.Now, form pretzels from the cheese dough and nicely shape it; then place it over a baking sheet.
8. 8.Sprinkle with a little bit of salt and bake for about 17 minutes.

Nutrition 113 Calories 2.5g Carbohydrates 0.8g Fiber

Cheesy Taco Bites

Preparation Time: 5 minutes

Cooking Time: 10minutes

Serving: 12

Ingredients

- 2 Cups of Packaged Shredded Cheddar Cheese

- 2 Tablespoon of Chili Powder

- 2 Tablespoons of Cumin

- 1 Teaspoon of Salt

- 8 Teaspoons of coconut cream for garnishing

- Use Pico de Gallo for garnishing as well

Directions:

1. 1.Preheat your oven to a temperature of about 350 F.
2. 2.Over a baking sheet lined with a parchment paper, place 1 tablespoon piles of cheese and make sure to a space of 2 inches between each.
3. 3.Place the baking sheet in your oven and bake for about 5 minutes.
4. 4.Remove from the oven and let the cheese cool down for about 1 minute; then carefully lift up and press each into the cups of a mini muffin tin.
5. 5.Make sure to press the edges of the cheese to form the shape of muffins mini.

6. 6.Let the cheese cool completely; then remove it.
7. 7.While you continue to bake the cheese and create your cups.
8. 8.Fill the cheese cups with the coconut cream, then top with the Pico de Gallo.

Nutrition 73 Calories 3g Carbohydrates 4g Protein

Nut Squares

Preparation Time: 30 minutes

Cooking Time: 10 minutes

Serving: 10

Ingredients:

- 2 Cups of almonds, pumpkin seeds, sunflower seeds and walnuts

- ½ Cup of desiccated coconut

- 1 Tablespoon of chia seeds

- ¼ Teaspoon of salt

- 2 Tablespoons of coconut oil

- 1 Teaspoon of vanilla extract

- 3 Tablespoons of almond or peanut butter

- 1/3 Cup of Sukrin Gold Fiber Syrup

Directions:

1. 1.Line a square baking tin with a baking paper; then lightly grease it with cooking spray
2. 2.Chop all the nuts roughly; then slightly grease it too, you can also leave them as whole
3. 3.Mix the nuts in a large bowl; then combine them in a large bowl with the coconut, the chia seeds and the salt

---

4. 4.In a microwave-proof bowl; add the coconut oil; then add the vanilla, the coconut butter or oil, the almond butter and the fiber syrup and microwave the mixture for about 30 seconds
5. 5.Stir your ingredients together very well; then pour the melted mixture right on top of the nuts
6. 6.Press the mixture into your prepared baking tin with the help of the back of a measuring cup and push very well
7. 7.Freeze your treat for about 1 hour before cutting it
8. 8.Cut your frozen nut batter into small cubes or squares of the same size

Nutrition 268 Calories 14g Carbohydrates 1g Fiber

Pumpkin & Banana Ice Cream

Preparation Time: 5 minutes

Cooking Time: 10 minutes

Servings: 4

Ingredients:

- 15 oz. pumpkin puree

- 4 bananas, sliced and frozen

- 1 teaspoon pumpkin pie spice

- Chopped pecans

Directions:

1. 1.Add pumpkin puree, bananas and pumpkin pie spice in a food processor.
2. 2.Pulse until smooth.
3. 3.Chill in the refrigerator.
4. 4.Garnish with pecans.

Nutrition: 71 Calories 18g Carbohydrate 1.2g Protein

JUICE AND SMOOTHIE RECIPES

Lucky Mint Smoothie

Preparation time: 5 Minutes

Cooking time: 0 minutes

Servings: 2

As spring approaches and mint begins to once again take over the garden, "Irish"-themed green shakes begin to pop up as well. In contrast to the traditionally high-fat, sugary shakes, this smoothie is a wonderful option for sunny spring days. So next time you want to sip on something cool and minty, do so with a health-promoting Lucky Mint Smoothie.

Ingredients

- 2 cups plant-based milk (here or here)

- 2 frozen bananas, halved

- 1 tablespoon fresh mint leaves or ¼ teaspoon peppermint extract

- 1 teaspoon vanilla extract

Directions

1. In a blender, combine the milk, bananas, mint, and vanilla. Blend on high for 1 to 2 minutes, or until the contents reach a smooth and creamy consistency, and serve.

VARIATION TIP: If you like to sneak greens into smoothies, add a cup or two of spinach to boost the health benefits of this smoothie and give it an even greener appearance.

Nutrition Calories: 152

Paradise Island Smoothie

Preparation time: 5 Minutes

Cooking time: 0 minutes

Servings: 2

Ingredients:

- 2 cups plant-based milk (here or here)

- 1 frozen banana

- ½ cup frozen mango chunks

- ½ cup frozen pineapple chunks

- 1 teaspoon vanilla extract

Directions:

1. In a blender, combine the milk, banana, mango, pineapple, and vanilla. Blend on high for 1 to 2 minutes, or until the contents reach a smooth and creamy consistency, and serve.

LEFTOVER TIP: If you have any leftover smoothie, you can put it in a jar with some rolled oats and allow the mixture to soak in the refrigerator overnight to create a tropical version of overnight oats.

Nutrition Calories: 176

Apple Pie Smoothie

Preparation time: 5 Minutes

Cooking time: 0 minutes

Servings: 2

This smoothie is great for a quick breakfast or a cool dessert. Its combination of sweet apples and warming cinnamon is sure to win over children and adults alike. If the holidays find you in a warm area, this smoothie may just be the cool treat you've been looking for to take the place of pie at dessert time.

Ingredients

- 2 sweet crisp apples, cut into 1-inch cubes

- 2 cups plant-based milk (here or here)

- 1 cup ice

- 1 tablespoon maple syrup

- 1 teaspoon ground cinnamon

- 1 teaspoon vanilla extract

Direction

1. In a blender, combine the apples, milk, ice, maple syrup, cinnamon, and vanilla. Blend on high for 1 to 2 minutes, or until the contents reach a smooth and creamy consistency, and serve.

VARIATION TIP: You can also use this recipe for making overnight oatmeal. Blend your smoothie, mix it with 2 cups rolled oats, and refrigerate overnight for a premade breakfast for two.

Nutrition Calories: 198

Choco-Nut Milkshake

Preparation Time: 10 minutes

Cooking Time: 0 minute

Serving: 2

Ingredients

- 2 cups unsweetened coconut, almond

- 1 banana, sliced and frozen

- ¼ cup unsweetened coconut flakes

- 1 cup ice cubes

- ¼ cup macadamia nuts, chopped

- 3 tablespoons sugar-free sweetener

- 2 tablespoons raw unsweetened cocoa powder

- Whipped coconut cream

Directions

1. 1.Place all ingredients into a blender and blend on high until smooth and creamy.
2. 2.Divide evenly between 4 "mocktail" glasses and top with whipped coconut cream, if desired.
3. 3.Add a cocktail umbrella and toasted coconut for added flair.
4. 4.Enjoy your delicious Choco-nut smoothie!

Nutrition 12g Carbohydrates 3g Protein 199 Calories

Pineapple & Strawberry Smoothie

Preparation Time: 7 minutes

Cooking Time: 0 minute

Serving: 2

Ingredients:

- 1 cup strawberries

- 1 cup pineapple, chopped

- ¾ cup almond milk

- 1 tablespoon almond butter

Directions:

1. 1.Add all ingredients to a blender.
2. 2.Blend until smooth.
3. 3.Add more almond milk until it reaches your desired consistency.
4. 4.Chill before serving.

Nutrition: 255 Calories 39g Carbohydrate 5.6g Protein

Cantaloupe Smoothie

Preparation Time: 11 minutes

Cooking Time: 0 minute

Serving: 2

Ingredients:

- ¾ cup carrot juice

- 4 cups cantaloupe, sliced into cubes

- Pinch of salt

- Frozen melon balls

- Fresh basil

Directions:

1. 1.Add the carrot juice and cantaloupe cubes to a blender. Sprinkle with salt.
2. 2.Process until smooth.
3. 3.Transfer to a bowl.
4. 4.Chill in the refrigerator for at least 30 minutes.
5. 5.Top with the frozen melon balls and basil before serving.

Nutrition: 135 Calories 31g Carbohydrate 3.4g Protein

Berry Smoothie with Mint

Preparation Time: 7 minutes

Cooking Time: 0 minute

Serving: 2

Ingredients:

- ¼ cup orange juice

- ½ cup blueberries

- ½ cup blackberries

- 1 cup reduced-fat plain kefir

- 1 tablespoon honey

- 2 tablespoons fresh mint leaves

Directions:

1. 1.Add all the ingredients to a blender.
2. 2.Blend until smooth.

Nutrition: 137 Calories 27g Carbohydrate 6g Protein

Green Smoothie

Preparation Time: 12 minutes

Cooking Time: 0 minute

Serving: 2

Ingredients:

- 1 cup vanilla almond milk (unsweetened)

- ¼ ripe avocado, chopped

- 1 cup kale, chopped

- 1 banana

- 2 teaspoons honey

- 1 tablespoon chia seeds

- 1 cup ice cubes

Directions:

1. 1.Combine all the ingredients in a blender.
2. 2.Process until creamy.

Nutrition: 343 Calories 14.7g Carbohydrate 5.9g Protein

Banana, Cauliflower & Berry Smoothie

Preparation Time: 9 minutes

Cooking Time: 0 minute

Serving: 2

Ingredients:

- 2 cups almond milk (unsweetened)

- 1 cup banana, sliced

- ½ cup blueberries

- ½ cup blackberries

- 1 cup cauliflower rice

- 2 teaspoons maple syrup

Directions:

1. 1.Pour almond milk into a blender.
2. 2.Stir in the rest of the ingredients.
3. 3.Process until smooth.
4. 4.Chill before serving.

Nutrition: 149 Calories 29g Carbohydrate 3g Protein

Berry & Spinach Smoothie

Preparation Time: 11 minutes

Cooking Time: 0 minute

Serving: 2

Ingredients:

- 2 cups strawberries

- 1 cup raspberries

- 1 cup blueberries

- 1 cup fresh baby spinach leaves

- 1 cup pomegranate juice

- 3 tablespoons milk powder (unsweetened)

Directions:

1. 1.Mix all the ingredients in a blender.
2. 2.Blend until smooth.
3. 3.Chill before serving.

Nutrition: 118 Calories 25.7g Carbohydrate 4.6g Protein

Peanut Butter Smoothie with Blueberries

Preparation Time: 12 minutes

Cooking Time: 0 minute

Serving: 2

Ingredients:

- 2 tablespoons creamy peanut butter

- 1 cup vanilla almond milk (unsweetened)

- 6 oz. soft silken tofu

- ½ cup grape juice

- 1 cup blueberries

- Crushed ice

Directions:

1. 1.Mix all the ingredients in a blender.
2. 2.Process until smooth.

Nutrition: 247 Calories 30g Carbohydrate 10.7g Protein

OTHER DIABETIC RECIPES

Seared Tuna Steak

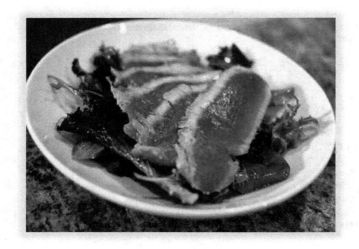

Preparation Time: 10 Minutes

Cooking Time: 10 Minutes

Serving Size: 2

Ingredients:

- 1 tsp. Sesame Seeds

- 1 tbsp. Sesame Oil

- 2 tbsp. Soya Sauce

- Salt & Pepper, to taste

- 2 × 6 oz. Ahi Tuna Steaks

Directions:

1. Seasoning the tuna steaks with salt and pepper. Keep it aside on a shallow bowl.

2. In another bowl, mix soya sauce and sesame oil.

3. pour the sauce over the salmon and coat them generously with the sauce.

4. Keep it aside for 10 to 15 minutes and then heat a large skillet over medium heat.

5. Once hot, keep the tuna steaks and cook them for 3 minutes or until seared underneath.

6. Flip the fillets and cook them for a further 3 minutes.

7. Transfer the seared tuna steaks to the serving plate and slice them into 1/2-inch slices. Top with sesame seeds.

Nutrition: Calories: 255Kcal Fat: 9g Carbohydrates: 1g Proteins: 40.5g Sodium: 293mg

Beef Chili

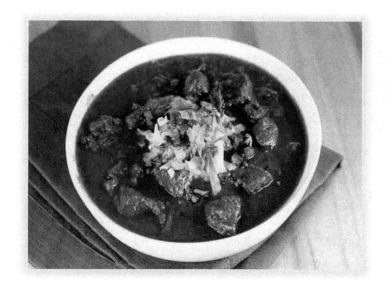

Preparation Time: 10 Minutes

Cooking Time: 20 Minutes

Serving Size: 4

Ingredients:

- 1/2 tsp. Garlic Powder

- 1 tsp. Coriander, grounded

- 1 lb. Beef, grounded

- 1/2 tsp. Sea Salt

- 1/2 tsp. Cayenne Pepper

- 1 tsp. Cumin, grounded

- 1/2 tsp. Pepper, grounded

- 1/2 cup Salsa, low-carb & no-sugar

Directions:

1. Heat a large-sized pan over medium-high heat and cook the beef in it until browned.

2. Stir in all the spices and cook them for 7 minutes or until everything is combined.

3. When the beef gets cooked, spoon in the salsa.

4. Bring the mixture to a simmer and cook for another 8 minutes or until everything comes together.

5. Take it from heat and transfer to a serving bowl.

Nutrition: Calories: 229Kcal Fat: 10g Carbohydrates: 2g Proteins: 33g Sodium: 675mg

Greek Broccoli Salad

Preparation Time: 10 Minutes

Cooking Time: 15 Minutes

Servings: 4

Ingredients:

- 1 ¼ lb. Broccoli, sliced into small bites
- ¼ cup Almonds, sliced
- 1/3 cup Sun-dried Tomatoes
- ¼ cup Feta Cheese, crumbled
- ¼ cup Red Onion, sliced

For the dressing:

- 1/4 cup Olive Oil
- Dash of Red Pepper Flakes
- 1 Garlic clove, minced
- ¼ tsp. Salt
- 2 tbsp. Lemon Juice
- 1/2 tsp. Dijon Mustard
- 1 tsp. Low Carb Sweetener Syrup

- 1/2 tsp. Oregano, dried

Directions:

1. Mix broccoli, onion, almonds and sun-dried tomatoes in a large mixing bowl.

2. In another small-sized bowl, combine all the dressing ingredients until emulsified.

3. Spoon the dressing over the broccoli salad.

4. Allow the salad to rest for half an hour before serving.

Nutrition: Calories: 272Kcal Carbohydrates: 11.9g Proteins: 8g Fat: 21.6g Sodium: 321mg

Cheesy Cauliflower Gratin

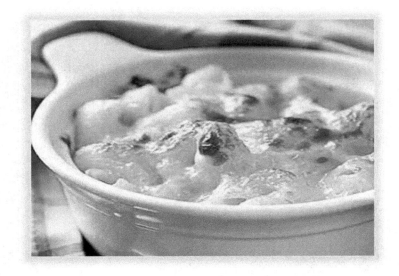

Preparation Time: 5 Minutes

Cooking Time: 25 Minutes

Servings: 6

Ingredients:

- 6 deli slices Pepper Jack Cheese

- 4 cups Cauliflower florets

- Salt and Pepper, as needed

- 4 tbsp. Butter

- 1/3 cup Heavy Whipping Cream

Directions:

1. Mix the cauliflower, cream, butter, salt, and pepper in a safe microwave bowl and combine well.

2. Microwave the cauliflower mixture for 25 minutes on high until it becomes soft and tender.

3. Remove the ingredients from the bowl and mash with the help of a fork.

4. Taste for seasonings and spoon in salt and pepper as required.

5. Arrange the slices of pepper jack cheese on top of the cauliflower mixture and microwave for 3 minutes until the cheese starts melting.

6. Serve warm.

Nutrition: Calories: 421Kcal Carbohydrates: 3g Proteins: 19g Fat: 37g
Sodium: 111mg

Strawberry Spinach Salad

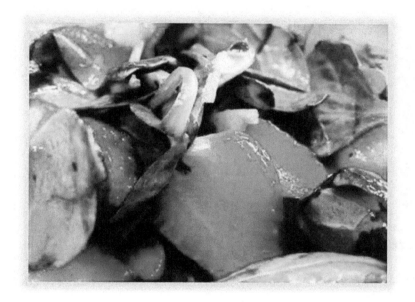

Preparation Time: 5 Minutes

Cooking Time: 10 Minutes

Servings: 4

Ingredients:

- 4 oz. Feta Cheese, crumbled

- 8 Strawberries, sliced

- 2 oz. Almonds

- 6 Slices Bacon, thick-cut, crispy and crumbled

- 10 oz. Spinach leaves, fresh

- 2 Roma Tomatoes, diced

- 2 oz. Red Onion, sliced thinly

Directions:

1. For making this healthy salad, mix all the ingredients needed to make the salad in a large-sized bowl and toss them well.

Nutrition: Calories – 255kcal Fat – 16g Carbohydrates – 8g Proteins – 14g Sodium: 27mg

Misto Quente

Preparation time: 5 minutes

Cooking time: 10 minutes

Servings: 4

Ingredients:

- 4 slices of bread without shell

- 4 slices of turkey breast

- 4 slices of cheese

- 2 tbsp. cream cheese

- 2 spoons of butter

Directions:

1. Preheat the air fryer. Set the timer of 5 minutes and the temperature to 200C.

2. Pass the butter on one side of the slice of bread, and on the other side of the slice, the cream cheese.

3. Mount the sandwiches placing two slices of turkey breast and two slices cheese between the breads, with the cream cheese inside and the side with butter.

4. Place the sandwiches in the basket of the air fryer. Set the timer of the air fryer for 5 minutes and press the power button.

Nutrition: Calories: 340 Fat: 15g Carbohydrates: 32g Protein: 15g Sugar: 0g Cholesterol: 0mg

CPSIA information can be obtained
at www.ICGtesting.com
Printed in the USA
BVHW090135040521
606354BV00005B/392